The Advanced Male Impotence Handbook

Latest Treatment Options for Managing ED, Master Your Mindset Enhance Performance with Proven Solutions to Restore Confidence and Boost Sexual Health Naturally

Erickson Tom Brown

Copyright

Contents

Introduction

A crucial component of human connection is intimacy, which includes emotional and physical ties that improve our quality of life. But for a lot of guys, the connection between intimacy and sexual health can be complicated by stigma, misunderstandings, and difficulties. Since it directly affects general well-being and quality of life, it is imperative to comprehend this relationship. Intimacy improves emotional wellbeing, builds stronger bonds with others, and makes life more satisfying when it thrives. The complex relationship between intimacy and sexual health is at the center of this investigation. The ability to have satisfying sexual interactions, feel at ease in one's body, and experience desire are all components of sexual health, which goes beyond the mere lack of illness or dysfunction. Men's sexual function, as well as their emotional and interpersonal dynamics, can be affected by problems like impotence, low desire, or anxiety. We can address these problems holistically and create more fulfilling relationships by acknowledging that sexual health is an essential aspect of intimacy. Male sexual health discussions are frequently veiled in secrecy despite the importance of these subjects. Many guys may struggle alone due to societal conventions and expectations obstructing candid communication.

Breaking this pattern requires creating a culture that normalizes and promotes conversations about sexual health. Men can be empowered to get the help they need, stigma lessened, and myths can be debunked via candid discussions. With an emphasis on the value of intimacy for general well-being, this e-book attempts to offer a thorough reference to male sexual health. We will examine ways to improve sexual health and rekindle intimacy through knowledgeable conversations, valuable techniques, and personal accounts. By working together, we can establish a culture of acceptance and understanding that enables men to confidently and resiliently embrace their sexual health journeys.

Description

Being in control of your sexual health is a continuous process that calls for bravery, openness, and a dedication to self-discovery. Understanding the relationship between physical and mental health can help you create a happy, passionate, honest, intimate life. Remember that the path to empowered intimacy is an ongoing experience rather than a final destination. You may handle the difficulties of sexual health with poise and confidence if you take proactive measures and welcome the help of loved ones and experts. Let your voice catalyze change in a society where discussions around male sexual health are frequently veiled in shame. Talk about your experiences, ask for help, and speak out for your needs. May you have the fortitude to pursue your goals and the fortitude to build solid and meaningful relationships as you go forward. You can restore your intimacy and sexual wellness. Accept it wholeheartedly and relish the great benefits that ensue.

Chapter 1

Introduction to Male Sexual Health

A fundamental understanding of anatomy and physiology is necessary to comprehend male sexual health, as is the demythologizing of prevalent myths and misconceptions that frequently skew conversations in this field. This chapter will cover both, setting the stage for a better-informed approach to sexual wellbeing.

Understanding the Male Reproductive System and Sexual

Understanding the parts of the male reproductive system and their functions is crucial to understanding male sexual health.

1. *The Anatomy of Male Reproduction*
Each of the multiple essential components that make up the male reproductive system

is vital to sexual health and function. The scrotum contains two tiny, egg-shaped organs called the testes. The testes produce sperm and testosterone, the main male hormone in charge of many sexual traits like libido and erectile function.

The coiled tube called the epididymis, located behind each testis, is where sperm develop and are kept until ejaculation. Sperm are transported by the muscular tube known as the vas deferens from the epididymis to the ejaculatory duct, where they combine with seminal fluid from the prostate gland and seminal vesicles to make semen.

The prostate gland and seminal vesicles produce fluids that nourish and transport sperm. The prostate produces the majority of the seminal fluid, which is especially important for ejaculation.

Penis: Made of erectile tissue, the penis facilitates semen production and sexual activity. Blood flow, nerve function, and psychological variables all affect one's capacity to get and keep an erection.

Scrotum: This skin pouch houses the testes and controls their temperature, which is essential for creating sperm. The scrotum modifies its posture to preserve ideal conditions for sperm viability.

2. *Sexual Response and Function*
It is essential to comprehend the physiological mechanisms behind sexual function. There are four stages to the male sexual response:

Excitement: This stage starts with psychological or physical stimulation, which causes the penis to get more blood and eventually result in an erection. During this stage, hormones like testosterone are important because they affect arousal and libido.

Plateau: Sexual tension increases during this stage. When the penis is completely erect, the Cowper's glands release pre-ejaculatory fluid, which balances the urethra's acidity and serves as a lubricant.

Orgasm: This stage ends with the release of semen, or ejaculation. Intense pleasure and pelvic muscular contractions are common symptoms of orgasm.
Resolution: The body gradually reverts to its resting state after an orgasm. There may be a refractory period during which

additional sexual excitement is momentarily impossible, and the penis loses its erection.

Myths and Misconceptions About Male Impotence

Many myths and misconceptions about male sexual health still exist despite advances in our understanding. These may result in false information, shame, and needless worry.

1. **Myth**: Only Older Men Are Affected by Erectile Dysfunction. Although it is more common in older men, younger men can still experience erectile dysfunction (ED). At any age, ED can be caused by a variety of factors, including stress, anxiety, depression, and lifestyle decisions (such as smoking and eating poorly). Younger guys are encouraged to ask for assistance without worrying about being judged when they realize this fact.

2. **Myth**: A Man's Masculinity Is Determined by His Sexual Behaviour. For many men, having sex is a sign of their masculinity. When problems develop, this harmful stereotype causes fear and embarrassment. In actuality, sexual prowess is not the only way to define masculinity; it is a complex concept. Emotional ties and healthy relationships are equally vital components of being a man.

3. **Myth**: Problems with Sexual Health Are Seldom Seen Sexual health problems are widespread, despite what the general public believes. Millions of men suffer from conditions like erectile dysfunction, low libido, and premature ejaculation. Recognizing the prevalence of these problems can lessen stigma, promote candid communication, and motivate people to seek help.

4. **Myth**: All Issues with Sexual Health Are Psychological Sexual health can be greatly impacted by psychological variables like worry and despair, but many problems have physiological causes. Sexual function can be affected by several conditions, including diabetes, cardiovascular disease, and hormone abnormalities. Men must understand the need to obtain medical advice to receive thorough care.

5. **Myth**: Sexual health problems cannot be treated. Many men think they are stuck with a sexual health problem once it occurs. Nonetheless, many efficient therapies are available, from medication to lifestyle modifications.
Men can take control of their sexual health by realizing that assistance is accessible.

Fostering a constructive and proactive approach to intimacy and general wellbeing requires an understanding of the fundamentals of male sexual health. By understanding the underlying anatomy and physiological processes, men can better appreciate their bodies and identify problems. Furthermore, dispelling widespread beliefs and misconceptions promotes healthy discussions about sexual health and empowers men to get the help they require without worrying about shame or stigma. Building on this foundation, we will examine lifestyle variables, psychological elements of sexual health, and doable tactics to improve overall sexual wellbeing and restore closeness as we proceed through this course.

Chapter 2

Warning Signs of Imminent Impotence

Men must recognize the warning signals of possible problems as they negotiate the complexities of sexual health. Many men may have periods of doubt about their sexual health, which several things, such as relational dynamics, emotional states, and physical conditions, can cause. This chapter explores the typical signs of sexual health issues and provides advice on when to get help from a specialist.

Recognizing the Symptoms
Recognizing Low Libido, Impotence, and Other Issues Sexual health problems can take many forms and can affect relationships, self-esteem, and general wellbeing. The first step to effectively treating these symptoms is understanding them.

1. Erectile dysfunction, or impotence
The inability to sustain or obtain an erection strong enough for sexual activity is the hallmark of erectile dysfunction (ED). Frequent incidents may point to a more serious problem, even though troubles may arise sometimes.

Symptoms include:

- Erection Difficulty

It can be upsetting and a symptom of underlying health issues when an individual struggles to get an erection during sexual excitement.

- Inconsistent Performance

Varying erectile firmness might be a sign of either psychological or physical issues.

- Loss of Morning Erections

Many men get erections on their own, whether they're sleeping or waking up. A discernible decrease in these incidents might call for more research.

2. Reduced Sexual Desire (Libido)
A decreased interest in sexual activity is referred to as low libido, and it can result from several factors, such as relationship dynamics, stress, or hormonal changes.

Symptoms Include:

- Reduced Interest in Sex

A discernible decline in sexual desire may impact intimate relationships and personal fulfillment. Disinterest in Intimacy: If you don't find physical intimacy with your spouse enjoyable or motivating, it could be a sign of emotional or psychological issues.

- Changes in Sexual Thoughts:

A lower frequency of sexual fancies or thoughts may be a sign of a more severe libido problem.

3. An Early Ejaculation

When a male ejaculates with little stimulation, usually before or soon after penetration, it is referred to as premature ejaculation.

Symptoms

- Lack of Timing Control

Regularly ejaculating earlier than intended can annoy and affect the quality of a relationship.

Feelings of Anxiety or Shame:

Premature ejaculation can cause anxiety and shame in many men, which can make personal relationships even more difficult.

4. Intercourse that hurts (dyspareunia) Pain during intercourse can be upsetting and needs to be addressed.

Warning signs:

- Physical Discomfort:
Genital pain during or after sexual activity may be a sign of underlying medical problems that need to be treated.

- Emotional Impact:
Anxiety about intimacy might result from experiencing pain during intercourse, starting a vicious cycle of avoidance.

Knowing When to Seek Professional Consultation

While identifying symptoms is essential, knowing when to get professional assistance is just as critical. Many men are reluctant to seek medical advice because they are embarrassed or afraid of being stigmatized, yet being proactive can have better results.

- Sustained Symptoms:
Getting aid is critical if you observe any previously listed symptoms continuing over

time. Recurrent ejaculatory problems, persistent low libido, or frequent erection difficulties are not just phase-related issues; they may indicate curable disorders.

- Mental Anguish:

Seeking help is crucial if problems related to sexual health are causing severe emotional suffering, such as anxiety, sadness, or relationship pressure. Sexual and mental health are linked, and taking care of one's emotional health can help one's physical health.

- Modifications to General Health:

See a healthcare professional if you've seen any changes in your general health, such as changes in weight, weariness, or long-term illnesses like diabetes or heart disease. These medical conditions should be thoroughly assessed since they have a direct impact on sexual function.

4. Relationship Stress:

It's critical to get help when sexual health problems start to negatively impact your relationship by causing avoidance, hate, or breaks in communication. Both parties can benefit much from therapy or counselling.

- Hormonal Changes Are a Concern:

Consult a healthcare professional if you suspect hormonal changes, such as decreased body or facial hair, gynecomastia (enlarged breast tissue), or noticeable mood swings. Sexual health can be greatly impacted by hormonal imbalances, which call for a professional assessment.

- Preventive Health Actions:

Maintaining sexual health requires routine check-ups with a healthcare professional, even in the absence of specific symptoms. Having proactive conversations about sexual function, lifestyle choices, and health exams might help spot possible problems before they become more serious. Effectively managing sexual health disorders begins with recognizing their symptoms. Men can take control of their sexual health by being aware of symptoms, including impotence, poor desire, early ejaculation, and painful intercourse.

We will go into further detail on lifestyle issues, psychological elements of sexual health, and doable tactics to improve intimacy and boost general well-being in the upcoming chapters. We can enable men to face their sexual health journeys with resilience and confidence by raising awareness and promoting preventative actions.

Chapter 3

The Psychology of Male Sexual Health

There is a strong correlation between sexual and mental health, with psychological variables having a significant impact on intimacy and sexual performance. This chapter highlights the need for emotional intelligence in creating wholesome relationships while examining how stress, anxiety, and depression can affect sexual function.

The Impact of Stress, Anxiety, and Depression on Sexual Performance

1. Fear:

Sexual health can be seriously hampered by anxiety, which can lead to a vicious cycle that is challenging to escape. For instance, performance anxiety can result in feelings of inadequacy, which can then cause libido loss or erectile dysfunction. Anxiety symptoms might include:

- Fear of Judgement:
Anxiety levels can be raised by worries about how a partner will interpret one's sexual performance, which makes it challenging to unwind and enjoy closeness.

- Physical Symptoms:
Without sexual context, anxiety can cause physiological reactions, including tense muscles, elevated arousal, and an elevated heart rate, all of which can impair performance.

Negative Thought Patterns:
A person who consistently thinks negatively about himself may find it challenging to participate completely in personal interactions, which may result in a complete avoidance of sexual encounters.

2. Depression:
Another psychological issue that has a significant impact on sexual health is depression. It may result in arousal issues, changes in energy levels, and a diminished interest in sex.

Essential Factors to Consider:

3. Loss of Interest:

Anhedonia, or the inability to feel pleasure, is one of the main signs of depression. When it comes to sexual desire, this might make closeness seem unattractive or unachievable.

4. Exhaustion and Low Energy:
Depression is frequently accompanied by a great deal of exhaustion, which might lower one's desire for intimacy and sexual engagement.

Problems with Body Image:
Depression can skew one's view of oneself, resulting in unfavourable sentiments about one's physical appearance, which can further impair sexual desire and performance.

3. Anxiety:
Regular stressors, such as those related to relationships, employment, or money, can also hurt sexual health. Stress can appear in several ways:

- Hormonal Changes:
Prolonged stress can raise cortisol levels, which can interfere with the creation of testosterone and reduce libido.

- Distracted Mindset:

Being present during intimate moments can be challenging, especially when dealing with stressful thoughts that are a barrier to closeness.

- Increased Tension:

Stress frequently causes physical tension in all parts of the body, which can affect how well a sexual encounter goes.

The Function of Emotional Intelligence:

Emotional intelligence (EI) is the ability to identify, comprehend, and control our emotions and those of others. Cultivating emotional intelligence can improve intimacy and sexual health.

1. **Self-Awareness**:

The foundation of emotional intelligence is self-awareness. You can gain a better understanding of how your emotions impact your sexual health by being aware of your feelings and responses. Important advantages include:

- Identifying Triggers:

You might try to proactively address the situations that cause anxiety or tension related to intimacy by determining what they are.

- Knowing Your Emotional Needs:

Awareness of your emotional needs makes expressing them to your partner more accessible, creating a more understanding and encouraging atmosphere.

2. **Compassion**:

Empathy—the capacity to comprehend and experience another person's emotions—is essential in close relationships. It is capable of:

- Improve Communication:

When both partners have empathy, they can talk about their thoughts and worries more honestly, which helps to avoid misunderstandings during private moments.

- Create Connection:

A more satisfying sexual connection may result from empathy's ability to fortify emotional ties.

3. **Good Communication**:

A healthy romantic life requires open and honest conversation about sexual needs and feelings. Effective communication techniques include:

- Using "I" Statements:

Using "I" statements to frame conversations (e.g., "I feel anxious when…") creates a more intimate and non-accusatory tone that facilitates understanding between partners.

- Making Time for Conversations:
Setting aside time to talk about intimacy outside of the bedroom allows partners to work through issues without feeling compelled to engage in sexual activity right away.

- Being Receptive to Feedback:
Promote an atmosphere where both partners are at ease discussing their emotions and experiences, enabling a reciprocal sharing of needs and wants.

4. **Creating Coping Mechanisms**:
The impacts of stress, anxiety, and depression on sexual health can be lessened, and emotional intelligence can be increased by cultivating good coping strategies. Methods could consist of:

- Meditation & Mindfulness:
Being attentive can help people stay in the moment, which lowers anxiety and improves sex.

- Therapy & Counselling:

Speaking with a mental health specialist can help you manage emotional difficulties and, in turn, improve your sexual health.

- Physical Activity:

Frequent exercise positively impacts sexual performance by lowering stress, elevating mood, and boosting self-confidence. Grasping and enhancing intimacy requires a grasp of the psychological components of sexual wellness. Stress, anxiety, and sadness can all be significant obstacles, but people can improve their relationships and deal with these issues more skillfully by developing their emotional intelligence.

As we proceed with our exploration of male sexual health, we will look at lifestyle choices that can promote mental and physical health and pave the way for a more satisfying romantic life. Men can restore their sexual health and develop closer relationships with their spouses by acknowledging the psychological aspects and practicing effective communication techniques.

Chapter 4

Factors that Affect Sexual Performance

Lifestyle decisions are crucial in the pursuit of restored closeness and strong sexual health. Sleep, exercise, and proper diet are not only elements of a healthy lifestyle; they are the cornerstones of sexual vigour. This chapter examines how these elements affect sexual performance and general health, offering tips for improving your relationships.

1. **Food and Supplements**:
When it comes to sexual health, the saying "you are what you eat" has a deep resonance. Our diets can either energize our bodies or make us feel lethargic. This section will examine important nutrients and dietary options to improve sexual function.

Zinc: The synthesis of testosterone and the general health of the reproductive system depend on this element. Zinc-rich foods, like chickpeas, pumpkin seeds, and oysters, can increase libido and promote sperm production.

Omega-3 Fatty Acids: Essential for erectile function, omega-3 fatty acids improve blood circulation and are present in fatty seafood like salmon and mackerel. Additionally, these good fats support cardiovascular health and lower inflammation.

Antioxidants: Antioxidant-rich foods, such as dark chocolate, almonds, and berries, help fight oxidative stress, which can have a detrimental effect on sexual health. Antioxidants also aid in maintaining healthy blood vessels to ensure proper blood flow during arousal.

2. Foods That Are Aphrodisiac

Some foods have been valued for their aphrodisiac qualities throughout history. Your romantic life can be energized by including these in your diet:

Dark Chocolate: Often referred to as the "food of love," dark chocolate has flavonoids that increase mood and circulation, strengthening emotions of closeness.

Avocado: Packed with vitamins, minerals, and good fats, avocados help boost hormone production and energy levels, making them the ideal accompaniment to a romantic dinner.

Spices: Add flavour and vibrancy to your food with ingredients like ginger and ginseng, which have been linked to better circulation and libido.

3. **Additional Resources for Assistance**

Supplements, in addition to a healthy diet, can improve sexual health. The amino acid L-arginine produces Nitric oxide, which improves blood flow and may support erectile function.

Maca Root: Known for its apoptogenic qualities, maca is a popular option for people looking to improve their sexual health because it may help balance hormones and boost libido.

Exercise

Exercise is a powerful remedy for mental and physical health. Regular exercise has a substantial positive impact on closeness, confidence, and sexual health.

Advantages of Frequent Exercise

Increased Blood Flow: Exercise increases blood flow, which is essential for sexual desire and erectile performance. Increased blood flow guarantees the body's ability to react to sexual stimuli. Increased

Endurance and Stamina:
Cardiovascular activities like swimming, cycling, or jogging increase stamina, allowing people to have more fulfilling personal experiences for longer periods.

Improved Body Image:
Consistent exercise increases body confidence and cultivates a sense of success. Increased libido and a willingness to participate in sexual interactions are directly correlated with feeling good about yourself.

Types of Exercises to Focus On

Strength Training:
Gaining strength through weightlifting increases testosterone levels, which can heighten sexual desire in addition to improving physical appearance.

- Exercises for Flexibility and Balance:

Yoga and Pilates, for example, increase flexibility, which enhances the comfort and enjoyment of physical closeness.

- Exercises for the Pelvic Floor:

Kegel exercises, frequently associated with women, can help males by strengthening the muscles in the pelvic floor. This improves erectile function and ejaculation control.

- Sleep and Recuperation:

The Impact of Good Sleep on Closeness and General Health Sleep is the rhythm that keeps us going smoothly in the complex dance of life. Good sleep is essential for optimum sexual health and is not merely a luxury.

Effects of Sleep on Our Sexual Health

- Hormonal Regulation:

Sleep is essential for controlling testosterone and other hormones. Reduced testosterone levels from sleep deprivation can have a direct effect on libido and sexual performance.

- Boost Mental and Happy Mood:

Getting enough sleep promotes mental clarity and a happy mood, which are necessary for close relationships. A lack of sleep can make you irritable and less interested in having sex.

- Recovery for Better Performance:
Men require good sleep to ensure their bodies are prepared for intimate interactions, just as athletes must recover to perform at their best.

How to Improve Your Sleep Quality

- Create a routine
Sleeping well involves regulating your body's internal clock by going to bed and waking up simultaneously every day.

- Establish a Calm Environment
Ensure your bedroom is peaceful, calm, and dark so you can sleep well. If necessary, consider using white noise machines or blackout drapes.

- Limit Screen Time
The hormone that controls sleep, melatonin, can be disrupted by the blue light that screens emit. Try to switch off electronics an hour or more before going to bed.

- Practice Mindfulness:
Including relaxation methods, such as deep breathing exercises or meditation, can help soothe the mind and prepare the body for a good night's sleep.

Lifestyle choices like sleep, exercise, and diet significantly influence male sexual health. By making thoughtful decisions in these areas, men can improve their sexual function, increase their confidence, and develop closer relationships with their partners. As we proceed with our exploration of male sexual health, we will examine the psychological facets of intimacy, stressing the significance of emotional intelligence and clear communication.

Chapter 5

Strengthening Emotional and Physical Connection

The balance between emotional and physical connection is crucial when it comes to sexual health. Partner intimacy involves open communication, trust, understanding, and physical affection. In addition to offering candid conversations about expectations, worries, and wishes, this chapter examines practical methods for strengthening emotional ties and physical affection.

How to Strengthen Emotional Connections and Physical Love with Your Partner

1. Making Quality Time a Priority
Emotional intimacy is fostered by providing opportunities for quality time spent together. Cooking, hiking, or spending a peaceful evening together are shared

hobbies, enabling partners to connect more deeply.

• Scheduled Date Nights:
Make time for one another regularly, away from outside distractions. This dedication to connection shows that the relationship is prioritized, which fortifies emotional bonds.

• Mindful Presence:
When together, practice being fully present. Put away phones and other distractions to foster an environment of complete focus.

2. Beyond Sex, Physical Affection
One of the most effective ways to develop intimacy is through physical contact. Feelings of intimacy are increased when non-sexual physical love is expressed.

• Cuddling and Holding Hands:
Small actions like holding hands while walking or cuddling on the couch foster comfort and warmth and strengthen emotional ties. Massage and Touch: Massages or soft touches can help partners relax and feel valued, boosting emotional and physical connection.

3. Verbal Expressions of Love:

Words have a tremendous amount of power to convey gratitude and love. Expressing emotions regularly can greatly improve emotional bonding.

- Affirmations and Compliments:
Please let your partner know how much you value their work, appearance, or other attributes. Affirmations boost self-esteem and strengthen relationships.

- Sharing Vulnerabilities:
By being honest about worries and fears, a safe environment may be established for both parties, which promotes intimacy and trust.

4. Taking Part in Common Experiences

Sharing experiences strengthens connections and creates enduring memories. Together, trying new things can rekindle interest and enthusiasm.

- Try New Things:
Whether going to a dance class, exploring new areas, or trying a new recipe, try new things together. Novelty can revitalize the relationship.

- Setting Goals Together:

Establishing common goals, whether related to fitness, vacation, or personal development, can strengthen the emotional connection and promote cooperation and unity.

Communication Skills

Effective communication is the foundation of any close connection. Strong communication skills help partners manage expectations and worries while expressing needs and wishes.

1. *Establishing a Secure Environment for Discussion*:
It is essential to create a secure space for candid discussion. It should be safe for both parties to express themselves without worrying about criticism.

- Pick the Correct Time:
When discussing delicate subjects, pick times when both partners are at ease and unhindered. Avoid starting significant conversations when you're under pressure.

- Employ Open-Ended Questions:
Promote discussion by posing open-ended enquiries that demand clarification. For example, rather than asking, "Did you enjoy last night?" Think about it: "How did our time together last night make you feel?"

2. *Engaging in Active Listening*
Active listening means paying close attention to what your partner is saying without interjecting. This method promotes comprehension and affirmation.

- Reflect and Clarify:

Reflect on what you've heard after your spouse expresses their opinions to ensure clarity. For instance, "It seems like you're worried about... Is that right?"

- Avoid Being Defensive:

Be open-minded when having conversations. Avoid getting defensive when your partner raises issues; try to grasp their viewpoint.

3. *Discussing Desires and Expectations*
Open communication about expectations and desires promotes intimacy and a closer bond between partners.

- Be Truthful About Your Needs:

Clearly state your sexual and relationship goals. Intimacy is strengthened by an open atmosphere fostered by honesty.
- Establish Mutual Boundaries:

Establishing mutual boundaries allows both couples to feel safe and respected, which can lead to satisfying intimacy.

4. *Resolving Insecurities and Fears*:
Fear and insecurity can hamper intimacy, yet resolving these emotions jointly can strengthen the bond.

Share Vulnerabilities: Discuss your anxieties about intimacy, performance, or the past. By sharing these vulnerabilities, partners might become closer and experience less loneliness.

- Encourage Supportive Reactions:

Partners should show empathy and reassurance in response to voiced concerns. This method creates a caring atmosphere where both parties feel appreciated. In conclusion, It takes deliberate work and honest conversation to strengthen emotional and physical ties. Partners can enhance their emotional ties by putting quality time, affection, and shared experiences first. When combined with successful communication techniques, these behaviours open the door to a more fulfilling and healthy intimate life. We will examine the psychological aspects of intimacy as we continue our discussion of male sexual health, emphasizing how to break down boundaries and improve the whole experience. Men can rekindle their sexual relationships and embrace a passionate and fulfilling journey together by cultivating emotional ties and encouraging candid conversations.

Chapter 6

Treatment Options for Male Impotence

There are numerous therapy options available for male sexual health issues, ranging from erectile dysfunction to diminished libido. This chapter overviews alternative medicines and medical interventions, highlighting their usefulness and efficacy.

1. Drugs

For men who are having problems with their sexual health, pharmaceutical medications are frequently the primary line of treatment. Here, we examine a few often prescribed drugs. These are the most well-known drugs for erectile dysfunction: phosphodiesterase type 5 (PDE5) inhibitors. Cialis (tadalafil), Levitra (vardenafil), and Viagra (sildenafil) all increase blood flow to the penis. Depending on the medicine, they can last anywhere from a few hours to a whole day and are only effective when sexual stimulation is provided.

Hormone Replacement Therapy (HRT):
HRT may be helpful for men who have low testosterone levels. Injections, patches, or gels can be used to give this medication, which helps to improve general sexual function, increase libido, and restore hormonal balance.

Alprostadil: This drug can be used as a urethral suppository or administered straight into the penis. It is helpful for people who might not react to PDE5 inhibitors since it relaxes blood vessels and increases blood flow.

2. Treatments

Concerns about sexual health can be addressed using a variety of therapy approaches in addition to prescription drugs:

Counselling and Psychotherapy:
For many men, psychological conditions like anxiety or depression are linked to problems with their sexual health. Relationship dynamics, self-esteem, and these underlying problems can all be addressed with the help of therapy.

Sex therapy: Trained professionals address sexual dysfunction and offer methods to enhance communication and closeness between partners. This method frequently incorporates exercises and behavioural techniques to boost self-esteem and lessen performance anxiety.

Pelvic Floor Therapy: The muscles involved in sexual function can be strengthened with pelvic floor exercises, which physical therapists frequently lead. This treatment is beneficial for men who have problems with erectile function or ejaculation.

3. **Medical Equipment**

Men with erectile dysfunction can benefit from several medical devices:

Vacuum Erection Devices (VEDs): These devices suck blood into the penis by creating a vacuum surrounding it, which makes an erection easier. The erection is then maintained during sexual activity by placing a constriction band at the base.

Penile Implants: Surgical procedures like penile implants may be considered for severe cases of erectile dysfunction that do not improve with other therapies. These gadgets can offer a long-term fix, enabling impromptu intercourse.

Alternative Therapies

The Function of Herbal Medicine, Acupuncture, and Holistic Methods Many men are turning to alternative therapies in search of all-encompassing solutions to issues related to their sexual health. These methods can improve general well-being and supplement conventional therapies.

- The use of acupuncture

Thin needles are inserted into predetermined body locations during acupuncture, which has its roots in ancient Chinese medicine. According to research, acupuncture may help with several sexual health concerns:

- Better Blood Flow:

Increasing blood circulation helps promote erectile function, and acupuncture may aid with this.

- Stress Reduction:

Acupuncture helps reduce stress and anxiety, which are frequent obstacles to sexual performance, by encouraging relaxation.

- Hormonal Balance:

According to specific research, acupuncture may have a beneficial effect on hormone levels, which could improve libido and sexual health in general.

Herbal Treatments

Traditionally, a variety of medicines have been used to increase libido and sexual performance. Despite differing scientific data, some well-liked choices are as follows:

- Maca Root:

Known as a natural aphrodisiac, maca is thought to increase energy and desire. It can be taken as a supplement or powder.

- Ginseng:

Often used in traditional medicine, ginseng is believed to increase stamina and energy, which may improve desire and sexual performance. Icariin, a substance found in Horny Goat Weed, may enhance blood flow and promote erectile function. Herbal supplements that focus on sexual health frequently contain it.

Holistic Methods

Holistic methods emphasize treating the patient as a whole, taking into account social, emotional, and physical aspects that impact sexual health. These could consist of:

1. **Mindfulness & Meditation**:

Practices that improve mental clarity and reduce stress can substantially impact sexual health by encouraging relaxation and emotional connection with partners.

2. **Dietary Adjustments**:

Promoting a well-rounded diet of fruits, vegetables, and good fats will help with sexual function and general health. Some foods, such as those high in omega-3 fatty acids and antioxidants, can be especially helpful.

3. **Lifestyle Changes**:

Sexual health can be significantly enhanced by cutting back on alcohol, stopping smoking, and reducing stress through hobbies or physical activity. Examining male sexual health treatment options involves a variety of methods, ranging from medications and therapies to complementary and alternative medicine and holistic practices. Men are more equipped to make decisions regarding their sexual health journey when they are aware of the variety of interventions that are accessible.

Chapter 7

Relationship Intimacy Challenges: Typical Problems and Solutions for Couples

Long-term partnerships may face difficulties that put their ties to one another to the test in the dance of love and intimacy. Couples can handle these dynamics gracefully if they are dedicated to knowing and connecting. This chapter examines typical intimacy issues in long-term relationships and provides sincere advice on restoring passion and romance.

1. Breakdown of Emotional Bonds:
The original spark that started a relationship might occasionally fade over time. Daily stressors, parenting obligations, and hectic schedules can gradually erode an emotional connection.

Solution: Purposeful Interaction Allocate specific, distraction-free time for each other.

This may be as easy as having a quiet evening at home or going out on a date once a week, which would provide time for meaningful discussions and laughing. Create an environment where emotional bonds can grow by participating in bonding activities like cooking or going for a walk.

2. Routine and Sexual Disinterest:

The excitement of intimacy may give way to routine as relationships get older, which can result in a decrease in sexual desire. Partners can find themselves slipping into a comfort zone that lacks the enthusiasm of their past.

Solution: Investigating Novelty as a Solution Incorporate spontaneity into your relationships. Try new things: change your routines, go to new places, or entertain new dreams. Even minor adjustments, such as adding music and candles to the atmosphere, can turn a routine evening into a magical retreat. Openly express your fantasies and enjoy the excitement of exploration with one another.

3. Breakdown in Communication:

Misunderstandings and unspoken emotions can damage intimacy. Partners may retreat if they feel alienated, which could result in more miscommunications. Open communication is the answer. Encourage open and sincere conversation. Plan frequent check-ins so that both parties can freely express their desires, feelings, and worries without fear of repercussions. Express ideas using "I" expressions to create an environment where everyone feels respected and heard. Saying something like, "When we don't spend quality time together, I feel distant," promotes connection rather than blame.

Techniques for Rekindling Romance in Relationships

1. Rediscovering One Another Partners may lose sight of the subtleties that initially drew them together amid life's hectic schedules. The partnership can be revitalized by rediscovering those attributes.

Solution: Share Memories. Spend time thinking about your shared experiences; go back to the locations where you fell in love, look through old photos, or talk about your favourite times. This trip back in time can remind you both of the love that still exists and rekindle the emotions that first drew you two together.

2. *Outside of the Bedroom, Physical Affection*

Intimacy on both an emotional and physical level is correlated. Emotional ties can be strengthened by increasing physical affection outside of sexual interactions. Daily Touch is the answer. Include small acts of affection in your everyday life, such as holding hands while walking, cuddling on the couch, or sneaking kisses in the kitchen. These deeds make more intimate encounters possible and lay the groundwork for warmth and connection.

3. *Surprise and Joy*

The thrill of romance can occasionally be tempered by routine. Introduce spontaneity to rekindle passion and desire in a relationship. Romantic gestures are the answer. Plan surprise date evenings, leave lovely notes in unexpected locations, or prepare their favorite dish on occasion to surprise your sweetheart. These little displays of affection remind you of your partner's place in your heart and express gratitude and consideration.

4. *Take Part in Adventures Together*

Exploring new things together can rekindle passion by kindling curiosity and excitement. The answer is to attend classes together. Consider signing up for a cooking lesson, dancing class, or painting night. Participating in shared activities breaks up the routine of everyday life and promotes teamwork by providing chances for connection and laughter.

5. *Put Intimacy First*
Prioritizing closeness conveys a strong message of love and dedication. Couples can develop stronger ties by intentionally fostering this area of their relationship.

Establish Rituals as a Solution:
Establish rituals honouring closeness, whether it's a typical date night, a weekend retreat, or a nightly practice sharing the day's highlights. These activities can establish a treasured place for connection and emphasize the value of intimacy in your lives.

Long-term relationships require patience and intentionality to navigate the nuances of intimacy. Couples can strengthen their ties and honour the eternal force of love by recognizing common problems and adopting techniques to reignite passion.

Conclusion

As we come to the end of our exploration of the complexities of male intimacy and sexual health, it is critical to acknowledge that each person possesses the capacity for empowerment. The anecdotes and observations presented in this book are a call to action and a guide.

Important Lessons for Empowerment

- Adopt Open Communication:

Discuss your expectations, worries, and desires openly with your partner. This conversation is essential to developing closeness, comprehension, and a stronger bond.

- Put Your Health First:

Invest in your physical and mental health by leading a healthy lifestyle, getting frequent checkups, and receiving the right treatments. Understand that caring for oneself is not selfish but essential to living a meaningful life.

- **Investigate Diverse Solutions:**

Keep an open mind to various therapeutic approaches, including natural and medical ones. Finding the method that works for you can improve your general quality of life and sexual health, as each strategy has advantages.

- **Develop Emotional Intelligence:**

You can be more empathetic and connect with your partner if you can comprehend and control your emotions. One effective strategy for fostering closeness and resiliency in relationships is emotional intelligence.

- **Rekindle Romance and Passion:**

Make an effort to find new ways to bring your relationship back to life. Making an effort to connect can change your private life, whether it be through romantic surprises, tiny acts of affection, or shared experiences.

www.ingramcontent.com/pod-product-compliance
Lightning Source LLC
Chambersburg PA
CBHW051848250726
48659CB00006B/2094